POCKET HEALERS
Ginkgo

BOOST BRAIN POWER & IMPROVE CIRCULATION

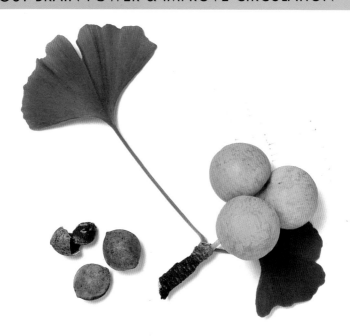

Stephanie Pedersen

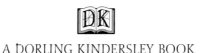

A DORLING KINDERSLEY BOOK

CONTENTS

HERBAL HISTORY

Long before over-the-counter medications and prescription drugs came on the scene, herbs proved to be powerful healers. Every culture on earth has used herbal medicine. In fact, herbal usage is older than recorded history itself: herbal preparations have been found at the burial site of a Neanderthal man who lived over 60,000 years ago.

When it comes to herbal medicine, many healing systems are available and useful. Perhaps the best known are ayurveda, Chinese medicine, and Western herbalism. Ayurveda is a system of diagnosis and treatment that uses herbs in conjunction with breathing, meditation, and yoga. It has been practised in India for more than 2,500 years. Ayurveda gets its name from the Sanskrit words *ayuh*, meaning "longevity", and *veda*, meaning "knowledge". Indeed, in ayurvedic healing, health can be achieved only after identifying a person's physical and mental characteristics (called "dosha"). Then the proper preventative or therapeutic remedies are prescribed to help an individual maintain doshic balance.

OTHER HERBAL HEALING SYSTEMS

Chinese medicine is another healing system that uses herbs in combination with acupressure, acupuncture, and qi gong. Sometimes called traditional Chinese medicine (TCM), this ancient system is thought to be rooted as far back as 2,800BC in the time of emperor Sheng Nung. Known as China's patron saint of herbal medicine, Sheng Nung is credited as being among the first proponents of healing plants. Chinese medicine attempts to help the body correct energy imbalances. Therefore herbs are classified according to certain active characteristics, such as heating, cooling, moisturizing, or drying, and prescribed according to how they influence the activity of various organ systems.

Many herbal practitioners believe that Western herbalism can trace its roots to the ancient Sumerians, who – according to a medicinal recipe dating from 3,000BC – boasted a refined knowledge of herbal medicine. Records from subsequent cultures, such as the Assyrians, Egyptians, Israelites, Greeks, and Romans, show similar herbal healing systems. But these peoples weren't the only ones using beneficial plants. The Celts, Gauls, Scandinavians, and other early European tribes also healed with herbs. In fact, it was their knowledge, combined with the medicine brought by invading Moors and Romans, that formed the foundation for Western herbalism. Simply put, this foundation formed a comprehensive system wherein herbs were grouped according to how they affected both the body and specific body systems.

After the discovery of the New World, Western herbalism was refined further with the benefit of wisdom gained from the American Indians, and the routine use of herbal remedies by physicians and for domestic use can be traced as far back as the 1600s. Herbs also featured heavily in medical pharmacopoeia until the 1900s.

However, with the creation of synthetic medicines in the 1930s interest in herbal medicines began to wane. New drugs were the great white hope for a disease-free future, but as time has passed they have been found to cause as many problems in terms of side-effects and contraindications as they solve.

Now, throughout Europe, America, and the world, gentler herbal remedies are enjoying a revival. What's been even more exciting is that many of the "folk" uses of these remedies have now been proven by science.

WHAT IS GINKGO?

Ginkgo has become a household word when it comes to herbs. Walk the aisles of any health store and you can't miss it: ginkgo in capsules, liquid extracts, tea, and more. Yet it is no medicinal newcomer – the herb boasts a long, distinguished history as an astringent, circulatory stimulant, expectorant and vasodilator. Over the centuries Chinese healers have used ginkgo to fight such wide-ranging ills as asthma, bladder infections, chronic coughing, headaches, memory problems, and premature ejaculation. Some of the earliest recorded usages of the herb – to expel phlegm, strengthen the lungs, and relieve wheezing – come from emperors who lived and worked before Christ was born, men such as Fu Si (2,953–2,838BCE), Shen Nung (2,838–2,698BCE) and Huang Di (2,697–2,595BCE).

Ginkgo biloba, commonly known as ginkgo, grows in Australia, Europe, and North America, but the tree is indigenous to China and its neighbouring countries. Extremely hardy, it thrives in a number of conditions including urban parks and pavement planters, polluted air, drought, and areas of low sunlight. It is so hardy, in fact, that it survived the Ice Age; archeologists have found fossilized ginkgo trees from the Triassic portion of the Mesozoic era, dated some 200 million years ago. Individual trees are capable of living nearly 4,000 years, and there are currently many 1,000- and 2,000-year-old ginkgo trees in China, Japan, and Korea.

Ginkgo leaves

A member of the Ginkgoaceae family, ginkgo is a deciduous tree that can reach heights of 37 metres (120ft). Its leathery, fan-shaped leaves turn gold in autumn, while the scented, apricot-sized fruits contain large seeds (also called "kernels" or "nuts"). In North America and Europe the tree's leaves that are used for medicinal purposes. Although the leaves are also utilized in Asia, the seeds and seed oil are more commonly used.

Today, ginkgo is best known as a brain function booster that is helpful in combating "cerebral vascular insufficiency illnesses", which are so common among the elderly of developed nations. These types of mental illnesses are caused by atherosclerosis of the cerebral arteries (thanks to rich diets heavy with animal fats) and include dementia, greatly impaired thinking, senility, short-term memory loss, and slowed mental response. Among the herb's compounds are flavone glycosides and terpene lactones, which work together to dilate blood vessels, increase blood circulation and inhibit coagulation. Together, these three actions encourage blood flow to the brain. How does all this aid mental function? When the blood flow to the brain is weakened, the brain's tissues receive less oxygen, which in turn impairs normal functioning. Increase oxygen-rich blood to brain tissues, and the brain functions better.

The herb also helps prevent or treat other illnesses produced by diminished blood flow, including impotence and leg cramping. Furthermore, the above-mentioned flavone glycosides and terpene lactones, plus the ingredient quercetin (which is an extremely potent-free radical scavenger), boast strong antioxidant, free radical-scavenging and membrane-stabilizing effects to help protect blood vessels, the brain, the eyes, and the heart against destructive free radicals.

· ALTERNATIVE · NAMES

Like many herbs, ginkgo is known by several names. Here are a few of them:

- Bai guo
- Ginkgo biloba
- Kew tree
- Maidenhair tree
- Silver apricot
- Yin guo
- Ying xing

HERBAL FORMULATIONS

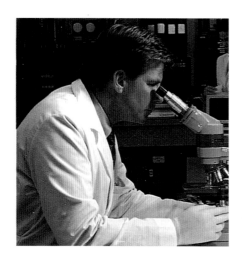

Researchers today perform thousands of rigorous clinical trials on the herbs sold in pharmacies and health stores. Most scientific studies with successful outcomes have used "standardized" herb formulations but the holistic approach is also currently finding favour. Standardized herb formulations means that particular therapeutic components are always present at specific concentrations. The benefit of standardization is that you will always be guaranteed a given potency but depending upon the method used to standardize, the full spectrum of constituents originally found in the herb might not be present in the final formulation. If all the components are present they are unlikely to be there in exactly the same proportions.

THE HOLISTIC APPROACH

Holistic herbal formulations, usually tinctures, contain the whole herb and their chemical composition will be as close as possible to the plant they derive from. Whole herb formulations may not always contain a consistent amount of active ingredients but manufacturers argue that it is the whole spectrum of ingredients, not just one or two active constituents, that determines the overall efficacy of the formulation. For advice on the most effective way to take specific herbs talk to a herbalist or pharmacist, or go to a reputable health store.

WHAT ABOUT GINKGO?

In the case of Ginkgo, the remedies that research has found to be most effective contain a high concentration of the active ingredients flavone glycosides and terpene lactones. Look for a product standardized to 24 per cent flavone glycosides and six per cent terpene lactone, with a recommended dosage of 100–150mg daily.

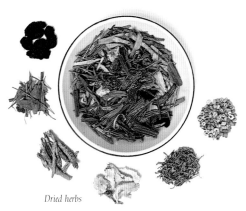

Dried herbs

· HERBAL BASICS ·

◆ Always follow the instructions on the label. Take the herb regularly and do not overdose.

◆ Don't expect instantaneous results. Some herbs may take a period of time to work.

◆ If you are pregnant don't take herbs without first seeking specific medical advice.

◆ Always check with your doctor if you are concerned that a herb may interact with a particular medication or be contraindicated by illness.

HERBAL LABELLING

You may have wondered why many herbal remedies don't give a clear indication of their potential use on the label. For example, you may be taking ginkgo to boost your memory, dong quai to help regulate your hormones, or St John's wort to lift depression but the packaging won't tell you that this is what the herb does. The reason is that only a proportion of herbs on the market are medically licensed: these are allowed to indicate their therapeutic uses but others, classified as normal foods, can't.

If a licensed formulation is available you may want to choose it instead of an unlicensed one because you can be sure that it contains efficacious ingredients and is made to the highest possible pharmaceutical standards.

UNLICENSED HERBS

Unlicensed herbal remedies are not necessarily any lower in quality. Most are made to the same reputable standards as licensed herbal formulations, and because they are technically "foods" they have to comply with strict food safety rules so that they do not harm human health. Getting a medical licence can take years, so it is no wonder that manufacturers produce herbal supplements without a licence to the highest possible standards.

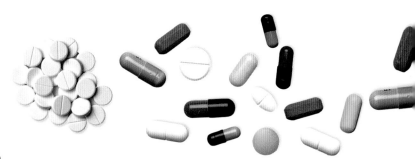

· MAKING THE BEST SELECTION ·

Whichever herbal supplement you chose, here are some guidelines:

◆ Choose a reputable manufacturer whose name you trust, or get advice from a herbalist or health professional.

◆ With tablets and capsules, compare doages carefully. Some manufacturers may mislead by claiming a powdered herb is an extract for example (an extract can be as much as 50 times stronger), or standardize herbs to a lower activity than other, more expensive, makes.

◆ Only choose herbal remedies that are properly sealed in tamper-resistant packaging and which have been clearly marked with a "best before" date. Check there is a contact address in case of any problem with the product.

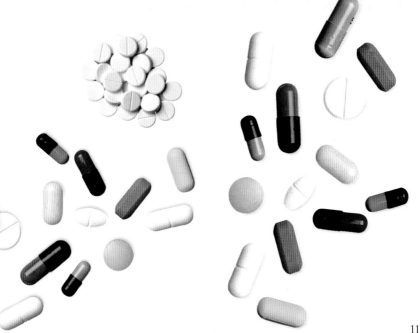

COMMON SIDE-EFFECTS

Like many medicinal herbs, ginkgo can cause mild side-effects.
Common side-effects can include:

DIZZINESS Though it is an extremely rare side-effect, a very small
number of individuals experience minor dizziness when taking ginkgo.

GASTROINTESTINAL UPSETS Ginkgo has been shown to cause
minor stomach upset in up to four per cent of individuals.

HEADACHE Though it is an extremely rare side effect, a very small
number of individuals experience mild headaches when taking ginkgo.

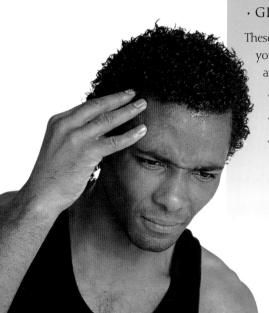

· GINGKO PRODUCTS ·

These are the forms in which
you will find gingko readily
available to buy:

- ◆ Tablets
- ◆ Powdered filled capsules
- ◆ Tinctures

AVOIDING RISK

◆ The doses in this book are generally aimed at adults. We strongly suggest consulting your child's doctor before administering ginkgo externally or internally. If your doctor does recommend ginkgo for your child, we generally recommend halving the adult doses suggested in this book. Again, please consult your child's doctor.

◆ Do not self-medicate with ginkgo while taking any type of anticoagulant medication. To do so can thin the blood too much, leading to possible internal bleeding. For information on how to safely switch from a synthetic anticoagulant to ginkgo, talk to your doctor.

◆ Do not self-medicate with ginkgo while taking any type of vasodilator medication. To do so can overdilate blood vessels. For information on how to safely switch from a synthetic anticoagulant to ginkgo, talk to your doctor.

◆ If you are pregnant, nursing, trying to conceive, or are taking any type of medication, please consult your doctor before taking ginkgo.

◆ To avoid any dangerous interactions between prescription medication and herbal medicine individuals with AIDS, cancer, a connective tissue disease, heart disease, kidney disease, liver disease, tuberculosis, or any other chronic illness should first consult their doctor before using any herbal formulation.

FORMULA GUIDE

Herbal remedies are sold in many different forms. Listed below are some of the most common products:

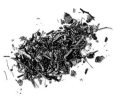

CAPSULES Capsules are usually made with gelatin and can be hard (made of two pieces, usually containing powders), or pliable (soft) and filled with liquid or paste. Two-piece capsules can also be pulled apart and the powder taken separately. Capsules usually contain fewer excipients (non-active) ingredients than tablets.

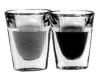

HERB, DRIED The flowers, leaves, stems and/or roots of many herbs are often available dried at health food stores and herbal pharmacies. While these are most commonly made into homemade teas, they can also be used to make decoctions, infused oils, sachets, etc.

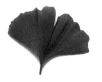

HERB, FRESH Herbs used in culinary and medicinal ways (such as parsley or dill) are most often found fresh. These can be made into homemade extract, juice, infused oil, tea, and more.

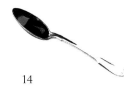

LIQUID EXTRACT (also called Extract). Macerated plant material is steeped over a period of time in a solvent or solvents such as alcohol, glycerin and/or water. The steeped liquid is then reduced to lessen the concentration of (or entirely remove) the solvents. Generally stronger than a tincture.

OIL, ESSENTIAL (also called Oil). Essential oils are the volatile oily components of herbs. They are found in tiny glands located in the flowers, leaves, roots and/or bark and are mechanically or chemically extracted. They are prescribed almost exclusively for external use.

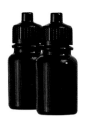

OINTMENTS Dried or fresh herbs are steeped in a base of oils and emulsifiers (such as beeswax, petroleum jelly or soft paraffin wax). After a period of time, the herbs are removed and the ointment packaged. For external use only.

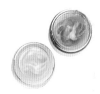

SYRUPS Syrups are generally a combination of herbal extracts and a sweetener, such as honey or sugar. Generally used for colds, flu, and sore throats.

TABLETS Tablets are made of all the relevant herbal and tabletting aids compressed using very high pressure. They are also relatively less expensive than comparable hard and soft gelatin capsules. Chewable tablets may be used for adult or child formulations.

TEAS/INFUSIONS Commercial herbal tea bags, loose dried, or fresh herbs are all available. This is a pleasant and acceptable way to take a herb, although to digest a useful quantity of the herb several cups have to be drunk daily.

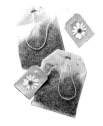

TINCTURES Tinctures are made by soaking plant material in a solvent – almost always alcohol – which is then pressed. Liquid from this pressing may be diluted with water before being packaged, usually in small dropper bottles. Tinctures are a very easy and pure way to take the herb.

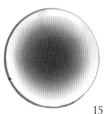

ASTHMA

SYMPTOMS Asthma is an inflammation of the airways and it is caused by an allergic reaction. Although not all sufferers are allergic to the same substances some common triggers are animal hairs, dust mites, mould spores, and pollen. When a trigger is inhaled, the body's antibodies react with the allergen producing allergen-suppressing histamine and other chemicals. Also, chest muscles constrict, the bronchial lining becomes inflamed, and the body creates more mucous, thus causing breathing difficulties, coughing (sometimes accompanied by mucus), painless tightness in the chest, and wheezing.

HOW GINKGO CAN HELP The ginkgolides in ginkgo have been shown in clinical studies to inhibit the chemical mediator that triggers allergic reactions. The herb's anti-inflammatory ability helps shrink swollen nasal and sinus linings so that allergy sufferers can breathe more easily.

DOSAGES For individuals who are in frequent contact with their "trigger allergen", ginkgo can be a preventative. Take 40mg of gingko extract three times a day before meals, or tincture as advised. For individuals who have infrequent contact with their allergen, up to 600mg of ginkgo extract can be taken an hour before anticipated contact.

RESPIRATORY ALLERGIES

SYMPTOMS A respiratory allergy feels similar to a cold – only with more itchiness. The condition is an immune-system response to a specific airborne allergen, usually animal hairs, dust, mould, or pollen. When the allergen is inhaled, an allergic person produces antibodies, which react with the offending substance and prompt the release of histamine. Histamine causes the lining of the nose, sinuses, eyelids and eyes to become inflamed, causing a variety of symptoms, including coughing, frequent sneezing, itchiness at the roof of the mouth, itchy eyes, itchy nose, itchy throat, runny nose, stuffy nose and watery eyes. Interestingly, when a person is allergic to pollen, the allergy is sometimes called hay fever, even though allergies to airborne animal hairs, dust, and mould produce identical symptoms.

HOW GINKGO CAN HELP The ginkgolides in ginkgo have been shown in clinical studies to inhibit the chemical mediator that produces allergic reactions. The herb's anti-inflammatory ability helps shrink swollen nasal and sinus linings so that allergy sufferers can breathe more easily.

DOSAGES For individuals who are in frequent contact with their "trigger allergen", ginkgo can be a preventative. Take 40mg of ginkgo extract three times a day before meals; or tincture as advised. For individuals who have infrequent contact with their allergen, up to 600mg of ginkgo extract can be taken an hour before anticipated contact with the trigger allergen.

CLAUDIFICATION (LEG CRAMPS)

SYMPTOMS When blood does not flow freely to the lower legs, painful cramps can develop, making it difficult to walk or stand. Called claudification after the limping Roman emperor Claudius, the condition occurs when the arteries leading to the leg become blocked with fatty deposits, or when the arteries' linings become inflamed. A diet heavy in animal fats is responsible in the first instance, while inactivity or smoking are generally to blame in the second.

HOW GINKGO CAN HELP In France and Germany ginkgo is routinely prescribed for claudification. A French study found that in 75 per cent of claudification patients, the herb increased blood flow to the lower legs. Two of ginkgo's constituents, flavone glycosides and terpene lactones, dilate inflamed or blocked arteries so that blood can reach the lower legs. In cases where claudification is caused by inflammation, these substances can also reduce swelling. Furthermore, the flavonoids that are in ginkgo help tissue regenerate by killing any free radicals created by lack of oxygen to the affected areas.

DOSAGES Take 40mg ginkgo extract three times a day with meals, or tincture as advised. Expect to begin seeing results after four weeks.

CORONARY ARTERY DISEASE

SYMPTOMS Coronary artery disease usually advances slowly over the course of years and even decades, but its impact can be instantaneous: in nearly a third of all cases, death occurs without any previous warning of the disease. Indeed, some people have no symptoms, while others may experience chest pain, constriction or a sense of heaviness in the chest, fatigue, pallor, shortness of breath, swelling in the ankles and/or weakness. Coronary artery disease occurs when cholesterol deposits build up on coronary artery walls. These special blood vessels provide oxygen and nutrients to the muscles of the heart. When they are unable to deliver adequate blood flow, the heart muscle begins to weaken, leading to angina (chest pain), congestive heart failure, and heart attack. When it comes to causes, a high-fat diet is most often implicated, although heredity, stress, inactivity, smoking, and alcoholism are also culprits.

HOW GINKGO CAN HELP Several studies have shown that ginkgo combats coronary artery disease in a number of ways. The antioxidant flavonoids help kill the artery-damaging free radicals created by cholesterol deposits. Flavone glycosides and terpene lactones dilate blocked arteries so that blood can reach the heart. These two elements also keep blood platelets from becoming sticky and thick; thin blood can pass more easily through blocked arteries.

DOSAGES If you are being treated for coronary artery disease do not take ginkgo without consulting your doctor.

HYPERTENSION

SYMPTOMS Hypertension, more commonly known as high blood pressure, is a condition in which blood travels through the arteries at higher pressure than normal. This increased blood flow literally wears out the blood vessels, heart, and kidneys and can lead to premature death. What causes hypertension? Cigarettes, alcohol, some medications, and certain illnesses can elevate blood pressure – but by far the most common cause of hypertension is clogged arteries from a high-fat diet. When blood vessels are blocked with fatty deposits, the heart must work harder to move the same amount of blood through them. This in turn increases the pressure at which the blood is pumped. Unfortunately hypertension is symptomless, leaving many individuals unaware that they even suffer from the condition until it is too late.

HOW GINKGO CAN HELP Flavone glycosides and terpene lactones work in two ways to treat hypertension: they dilate blood vessels so that blood can more easily pass through; and they inhibit coagulation so that blood does not clog on deposits as it moves through the veins.

DOSAGES Whilst ginkgo has the potential to prevent and treat high blood pressure, it is important not to self-medicate for this condition. Take ginkgo for hypertension only under the supervision of a qualified medical practitioner.

· GINKGO AND CHINESE MEDICINE ·

In traditional Chinese medicine ginkgo is used to treat illnesses caused by "damp heat", deficient "kidney yin", or deficient "lung qi". Below is a summary of what kinds of illnesses these are:

◆ Damp heat imbalances often appear as skin conditions. Abscesses, boils, chicken pox, herpes, infected sores, lesions, and shingles are examples. Internal damp heat conditions involve the upper respiratory tract.

◆ Deficient kidney yin can cause a dry mouth and throat, excessive thirst, flushed skin, hot hands and feet, insomnia, lower-back pain, night sweats, ringing in the ears, or premature ejaculation.

◆ Deficient lung qi is characterized by the following: allergies, asthma, chills, general weakness, shallow cough, shallow respiration, sparse white phlegm, susceptibility to colds, sweating, weak or soft voice.

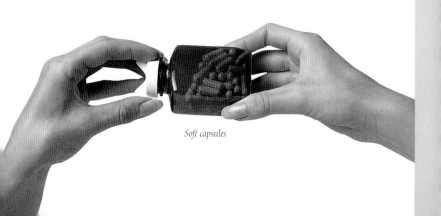

Soft capsules

TINNITUS

SYMPTOMS Individuals with tinnitus hear noise in one ear – usually buzzing, hissing, ringing, roaring or whistling – when no such noise is present in the environment. These noises may be continuous or intermittent, they may or may not be synchronized with the heartbeat, they may range from soft to loud, and they may be accompanied by hearing loss. Tinnitus is usually a secondary symptom of a variety of conditions, including acoustic trauma, Ménière's disease, middle ear infection, occupational hearing loss, or a build-up of wax. Sometimes, however, tinnitus can occur spontaneously with no explanation.

HOW GINKGO CAN HELP In French studies ginkgo has been shown to lessen or eradicate tinnitus. It is believed that the herb works in three ways: improving blood circulation to the ear; strengthening nerve connections between the ear and brain; and fighting off age-related free radicals that can damage nerve cells in the ear.

DOSAGES Take 40mg ginkgo extract three times a day with meals, or tincture as advised. Expect to see mild results within two weeks, stronger results in six to eight weeks.

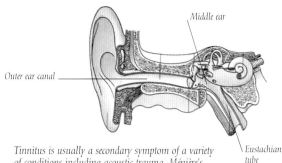

Middle ear

Outer ear canal

Eustachian tube

Tinnitus is usually a secondary symptom of a variety of conditions including acoustic trauma, Ménière's disease, middle ear infection, occupational hearing loss, or a build-up of wax.

· GINKGO AROUND THE WORLD ·

To the Germans and French, ginkgo is a highly regarded treatment for Alzheimer's disease, depression, circulatory disorders, hearing problems and memory loss. It is so highly regarded, in fact, that 1.5 million prescriptions for the herb are written every week. In Germany, the herb accounts for one per cent of all prescription medication, while in France it accounts for four per cent.

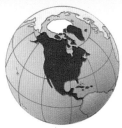

AGE-RELATED MACULAR DEGENERATION

SYMPTOMS Also known as involutional macular degeneration or senile degeneration, this is the most frequent cause of legal blindness in the US and the UK. The macula, which is the central portion of the retina, is responsible for central vision. As some people age, however, the layer of insulation between the retina and the blood vessels behind it begins to break down, making it easy for fluid to leak into the retina from the blood vessels. As a result of this damage, scar tissue begins to form on the macula, creating a corresponding blind spot. This scar tissue begins to spread, thus creating an increasingly larger blind area in an individual's field of vision. While a person's peripheral vision is largely unaffected, it becomes more difficult for the individual to see what lies straight ahead. Experts believe that damage done by free radicals is what causes age-related macular degeneration.

HOW GINKGO CAN HELP Ginkgo is regularly used in France and Germany as a treatment for macular degeneration. A French study of patients with macular degeneration proved ginkgo was successful in improving central vision; the herb's flavonoids help reverse free radical damage, which is believed to cause macular degeneration.

DOSAGES Studies have shown that once 20 per cent or more of a person's vision is lost to macular degeneration, that vision cannot be returned. For this reason, consider taking ginkgo has a preventative formulation: take 40mg ginkgo extract three times a day with meals, or tincture as advised.

If you already have signs of macular degeneration, you can diminish or prevent any further damage by taking two doses of 40mg ginkgo extract three times a day with meals, or tincture as advised.

· GINKGO: ANTI-AGING MEDICATION? ·

In medical circles, one of the most famous studies on ginkgo was conducted in France and published in the September 1986 issue of La Presse Médicale. French researchers examined 166 geriatric patients in 17 areas: ability to walk, appetite, anxiety, cooperation, depression, disturbances in orientation, emotional stability, fatigue, headache, initiative, personal care, ringing in the ears, short-term memory, sleep abnormalities, sociability, vertigo, and vivacity. After taking 160mg of ginkgo every day for three months, all test subjects – regardless of their original state – made mild to excellent improvement in all 17 areas.

Ginkgo may improve your body's well-being.

HAEMORRHOIDS

SYMPTOMS Just under the membrane lining the lowest part of the anus and rectum are clusters of veins. Sometimes these veins become swollen – perhaps as a result of pregnancy, chronic constipation, or straining during a bowel movement. These swollen veins are called haemorrhoids. Symptoms of the condition can include anal itching, tenderness (especially during a bowel movement), protrusion of soft tissue at the anus and bright red blood on toilet paper or stool after a bowel movement.

HOW GINKGO CAN HELP A French study found that ginkgo was effective in lessening symptoms of acute and chronic haemorrhoids in 86 per cent of patients. Ginkgo has powerful anti-inflammatory abilities that can reduce the swelling that causes haemorrhoids.

DOSAGES Apply ginkgo fomentation directly to affected area up to three times a day, or swab the area up to three times a day with ginkgo tea. Taken internally, ginkgo also helps shrink haemorrhoids. Take 40mg ginkgo extract three times a day with meals, or tincture as advised. Discontinue when haemorrhoid has healed. Pregnant women should not take ginkgo for haemorrhoids without medical advise.

· USING MORE THAN THE LEAVES ·

Western research and usage has concentrated solely on the
ginkgo leaf, and so most of the formulations mentioned in this
book focus only on the leaf. However, in China, Korea, and
Japan doctors use ginkgo seeds for complaints linked to "wind-
damp" illnesses. These ailments include allergies, asthma, bladder
infections, blisters, boils, chills, colds, fever, heaviness in the chest,
heaviness in the head, influenza, joint pain, muscle cramps, skin
rashes, sparse urination, tuberculosis, and uterine cramps. The
seeds, which are mildly toxic in their raw state, are boiled and
dried. They can be ground and taken as a powder or swallowed
in capsule form, but more often they are left whole and eaten
alone or added to food. Because the plum-like fruit encapsulating
the seeds can cause a poison-ivy-like rash, gloves should be
worn while harvesting. Tins of ginkgo seeds can be bought
in most Chinese supermarkets; the kernels are often added to
recipes. For more information on using ginkgo
seeds, please contact a qualified doctor of
Chinese medicine.

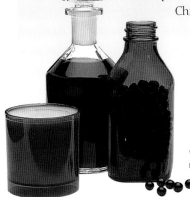

*Various herbal
remedies*

IMPOTENCE

SYMPTOMS While anything from too much alcohol to anger or depression can cause short-term erectile problems, impotence is defined as a chronic inability to have or sustain an erection. In 90 per cent of cases an organic cause is the culprit, which usually means that the blood flow leading from the heart to the penis is diminished by fatty deposits in the arteries.

HOW GINKGO CAN HELP In Chinese medicine ginkgo is regularly prescribed to treat impotence. Indeed, several American studies of impotent men have found ginkgo effective in restoring blood flow to the penis, thereby helping patients to achieve and maintain erections. The herb does this by dilating blood vessels, thus allowing blood to reach the penis more easily. In rare cases impotence is caused by low levels of testosterone, which is produced in the testes. Overall glandular functions are controlled by the pituitary.

DOSAGES Take 40mg ginkgo extract three times a day with meals, or tincture as advised. Expect to see results in six to eight weeks.

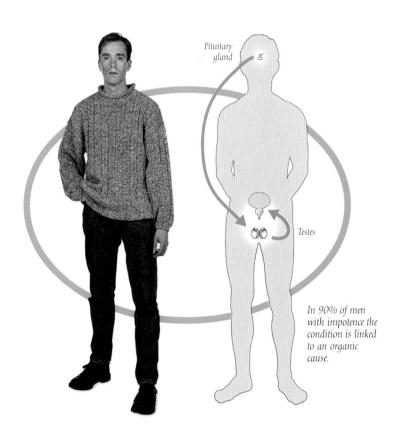

Pituitary gland

Testes

In 90% of men with impotence the condition is linked to an organic cause.

ALZHEIMER'S DISEASE

SYMPTOMS Alzheimer's disease primarily strikes older adults, most commonly affecting those aged 65 and older, although it can strike people in their 40s or 50s. In fact, almost one in 10 people over the age of 65 is diagnosed with Alzheimer's. Alzheimer's is an incurable disease that destroys brain cells – usually those of the cerebral cortex – causing dementia. Symptoms appear progressively, usually in the following order: forgetfulness, shortened attention span, disintegration of personality, disorientation, memory loss, confusion, restlessness, inability to read, wandering, lack of patience, loss of impulse control, inappropriate behaviour, aggressiveness, irritability, swearing, lack of coordination, delusions, hallucinations, loss of language, lack of bladder and bowel control, and inability to feed oneself. Currently, there is no diagnostic test for Alzheimer's; the most foolproof test for the disease is an autopsy to examine brain tissue. That said, doctors can make an accurate diagnosis in up to 90 per cent of all cases after a careful medical history and physical examination. It's not known exactly what causes Alzheimer's. Some researchers believe it is an inflammatory response to infection; others blame it on free radicals, environmental toxins, or lack of blood flow to the brain. Whatever the culprit, genetics is often a factor.

HOW GINKGO CAN HELP At present there is no cure for Alzheimer's disease, although several studies have shown that ginkgo can delay the onset of the disease or lessen its severity. In a recent German study, 216 patients with mild to moderate Alzheimer's disease were divided into two groups. One group received 240mg of ginkgo a day; the other group received a placebo. At the end of one month, the group taking ginkgo showed increased mental alertness and decreased irritability, while the placebo group remained the same. Other studies have shown that if Alzheimer's patients take ginkgo for between four and eight weeks they have an increase in the turnover of norepinephrine (an important chemical transmitter) in the brain, indicating increased brain activity.

DOSAGES Take 40mg of gingko extract three times a day before meals; or tincture as advised. Expect to see results after four weeks.

· DEMENTIA VS. ALZHEIMER'S DISEASE ·
– WHAT'S THE DIFFERENCE?

The word "dementia" refers to a gradual loss of mental functioning, regardless of its cause. Dementia is not a disease but a syndrome, meaning it is characterized by a group of symptoms that can include a gradual loss of short-term memory, inability to learn new information, growing tendency to repeat oneself, misplacing objects, confusion, getting lost, slow disintegration of personality, loss of judgement, lack of social graces, increasing irritability, restlessness and lack of bowel and/or bladder function. Alzheimer's, on the other hand, is actually a disease – a disease that causes dementia. Other conditions that can produce dementia are Huntington's disease, multiple sclerosis, Parkinson's disease, AIDS, strokes, and brain damage caused by trauma.

DEPRESSION

SYMPTOMS The condition often begins with no apparent trigger, though it can also develop from a specific incident. Symptoms can include a change in appetite, decreased self-esteem, grief, helplessness, impaired daily functioning, irritability, the loss of interest in once-enjoyable activities, inappropriate guilt, lethargy, neglect of physical appearance, malaise, self-reproach, a sense of doom, sleep disturbances, slowed physical and mental responses, social withdrawal and even thoughts of suicide.

HOW GINKGO CAN HELP The German Ministry of Health Committee for Herbal Remedies approves ginkgo for improving mood and mental processes, and several German studies have found ginkgo to be an effective anti-depressant. In fact, one study found that a group of individuals aged between 51 and 78 who had not responded to pharmaceutical anti-depressants showed marked improvement after four weeks when given 240mg of ginkgo extract daily. The herb helps combat depression in two ways: by increasing blood flow to the brain for more efficient brain functioning; and by increasing brain levels of dopamine. Dopamine, a neurotransmitter, helps to regulate moods and is critical to the transfer of information among nerves.

DOSAGES Take 40mg of gingko extract three times a day before meals; or tincture as advised. Expect to see mild results within two weeks, and stronger results in four to eight weeks.

· RADIATION ·

Ginkgo contains a group of ingredients known as flavonoids, of which the major ones are quercetin, kaempferol, and isorhamnetin. These substances are intense antioxidants, able to fight off the most aggressive onslaught of free radicals. This is why it is sometimes used by scientists to counteract the effects of radiation. One of the most celebrated examples of this came after the 1987 malfunction of the Chernobyl nuclear power plant in Russia. Researchers studied 30 workers responsible for dismantling the plant and cleaning up the toxic waste. Exposure to nuclear radiation had left each individual with greatly damaged chromosomes, which in turn put the group at high risk for cancer. In an effort to administer a treatment free of side-effects, doctors decided upon ginkgo. Each worker received 40mg of ginkgo extract three times a day. At the end of two months, all were found to have greatly normalized chromosomes.

Ginkgo may normalize damaged chromosomes in the body.

IMPAIRED CONCENTRATION

SYMPTOMS Weakened concentration is often associated with ageing – and with good reason. Individuals who have spent a lifetime eating a diet heavy in animal products often have cerebral arteries that have become hardened and coated with plaque. The result: less oxygen-rich blood is able to reach the brain. Without this nourishment, a number of the brain's mental functions can become impaired, concentration included. However, clogged blood vessels aren't the only cause of impaired concentration. Younger individuals who are besieged by stress, or are inactive, sleep-deficient, or drink heavily – all of which can temporarily slow blood flow to the brain – can also suffer from reduced concentration. Regardless of the cause, impaired concentration is characterized by an inability or reduced ability to concentrate during conversations and lectures and difficulty focusing on work tasks and written material.

HOW GINKGO CAN HELP Flavone glycosides and terpene lactones work together to dilate blood vessels, increase blood circulation and inhibit blood coagulation. Together, these three actions encourage blood flow to the brain for improved mental functioning.

DOSAGES Take 40mg of gingko extract three times a day before meals; or tincture as advised. Expect to see mild results within two weeks, stronger results in six to eight weeks.

The ability to concentrate decreases when individuals of any age have more stress than they can handle, drink heavily, and do not get enough physical exercise or sleep.

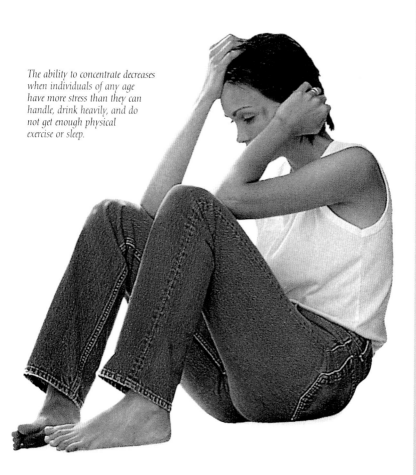

IMPAIRED SHORT-TERM MEMORY

SYMPTOMS Memory is a complex process that we still don't completely understand. Why is it that, as we age, we often become even more forgetful of things that have just occurred? Scientists are not sure exactly what lies behind these temporary glitches in our memory banks. They know, however, that many older individuals have experienced a lifetime of fat-heavy meals, resulting in hardened, plaque-coated cerebral arteries, reducing the amount of oxygen-rich blood to the brain. Without this nourishment, a number of the brain's mental functions can become impaired, memory included. However, clogged blood vessels are not the only cause. Younger individuals who are besieged with stress, are inactive, sleep-deficient, or drink heavily, can also suffer from impaired short-term memory due to a temporarily slow blood flow to the brain.

HOW GINKGO CAN HELP Bulgarian, English, French, and German researchers have all conducted separate studies that show ginkgo to be helpful in combating reduced short-term memory. The constituents flavone glycosides and terpene lactones work together to dilate blood vessels, increase blood circulation, and inhibit blood coagulation. Together, these three actions encourage blood flow to the brain for improved mental functioning.

DOSAGES Take 40mg of gingko extract three times a day before meals; or tincture as advised. Expect to see mild results within two weeks, stronger results in six to 12 weeks.

· MEMORY AID ·

Taking a ginkgo formulation can help with revision or memorizing a speech, for example. In French studies of short-term usage, ginkgo was found to be safe, effective, and without side-effects when taken at a high dosage (600mg) one hour before studying. Although lower dosages (120mg and 240mg) are routinely prescribed for permanent memory impairment, these quantities were shown to be ineffective when used as a temporary study aid. That said, high dosages of ginkgo daily should not be taken for long periods of time. While studies have yet to uncover any hazards, there is the remote possibility that long-term, elevated daily doses of ginkgo can thin the blood to unhealthy levels. Instead, limit 600mg doses to an occasional weekly study session. To further maximize your ability to absorb information, do not study when tired or hungry, and avoid studying in noisy environments. Experts say that brain power can be boosted by breaking up study periods into blocks of 20-40 minutes before stopping for a 10 minute rest and then returning to spend 10 minutes reviewing what has already been learned.

Migraine Headaches

SYMPTOMS Also called vascular headaches, migraines are extremely painful headaches that occur when cerebral blood vessels constrict, thus allowing less blood to reach the brain. The one constant symptom is severe head pain – often so extreme that individuals can become nauseated and vomit. The pain typically begins on one side of the head and may gradually spread and throb. Migraines are usually preceded by several warning signals. Between two to eight hours before a migraine occurs some people may experience elation, drowsiness, intense thirst, irritability, and a craving for sweets. About 15–30 minutes before the migraine occurs, some people may see an "aura": a group of symptoms that can include blank spots within the field of vision, dizziness, sparkling flashes of light, temporary numbness or paralysis of one side of the body, and zigzag lines that cross the field of vision. It is not known why some people get migraines, although stress, alcohol consumption, specific foods, and oral contraceptives can trigger cerebral vessels to constrict in some individuals, causing vascular headaches.

HOW GINKGO CAN HELP Ginkgo is a vasodilator, dilating constricted blood vessels so that blood can flow smoothly. Studies have shown that ginkgo's vasodilating action helps to relieve migraines.

DOSAGES For individuals who suffer from frequent migraines, ginkgo can be a preventative when 40mg of gingko extract is taken three times a day before meals, or tincture taken as advised.

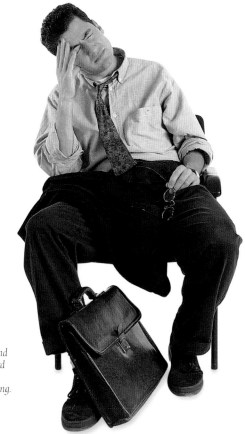

Migraines can last anything from two hours to two days and are often accompanied by disturbances of vision and/or vomiting.

Premenstrual Syndrome

Symptoms Premenstrual syndrome, popularly known as PMS, is a predictable pattern of physical and emotional changes that occur in some women just before menstruation. Symptoms can be barely noticeable or extreme and include abdominal swelling, anxiety, bloating, breast soreness, clumsiness, depressed mood, difficulty concentrating, fatigue, fluid retention, headaches, irritability, lethargy, skin eruptions, sleep disturbances, swollen hands and feet, and weight gain.

How Ginkgo Can Help Several American and French studies have shown that ginkgo's anti-inflammatory powers help to reduce the swelling, breast soreness, and fluid retention associated with PMS. Furthermore, the herb combats headaches by boosting blood circulation to the brain.

Dosages Two weeks before your period, begin taking 40mg of gingko extract three times a day before meals, or tincture as advised. Discontinue on the second day of menstruation. It can be used this way on a monthly basis. For temporary relief from discomfort and irritability, try a cup of ginkgo tea.

· PMS FACTS ·

Studies have shown that women who regularly consume three or more cups of coffee daily are four times more likely than non or moderate coffee drinkers to have severe PMS.

◆ A significant number of PMS sufferers also have some type of thyroid dysfunction.

◆ Recent research suggests that some women who suffer from PMS may be deficient in melatonin, a hormone that regulates the body's biological clock. Melatonin is secreted at night by the pineal gland.

◆ In Japan, women suffering from the effects of PMS drink kombuchu tea. This energizing beverage is high in antioxidants and immune-boosting phytochemicals.

◆ Many gynaecologists recommend oral contraceptives for women with PMS. Oral contraceptives lessen PMS symptoms by "tricking" the body into believing it is pregnant.

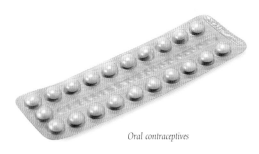

Oral contraceptives

GROW IT YOURSELF

The ginkgo tree is an amazingly hardy breed, displaying attractive fan-shaped, medium-green foliage and plum-like fruit. If you would like to try growing this eye-catching tree yourself, be aware that it is slow-growing, often taking up to 20 years to reach 6-9 metres (20-30ft).

GINKGO BILOBA

SIZE Up to 37 metres (120ft) high.

NATIVE HABITAT Dry, sunny to partially shady areas of China. It has been introduced to Australia, Europe, Korea, Japan, India, and the US, where it often thrives in urban parks.

Gingko leaves help to improve the body's circulation.

CULTIVATION Well adapted to poor, dry soil and polluted environments. Young ginkgo trees can be purchased from nurseries. Choose a preferably sunny, or partially sunny, area of your garden and plant the tree in mid- to late-spring after the last frost. Water sparingly and do not prune or fertilize the plant for the first year. The tree should grow 15-30 centimetres (6-12in) in the first year. A limited amount of leaves can be harvested at the end of the second summer.

Note: *If you intend to harvest the ginkgo leaves for medicinal purposes, do not treat the tree with pesticides.*

GATHERING YOUR OWN

Hunting wild herbs is a satisfying introduction to herbal therapy but when done thoughtlessly it can cause plant extinction. In fact, today's increased interest in wild herb gathering has left many indigenous plants extinct; echinacea, ginger, ginseng, goldenseal, sweet grass, and wild carrot are now nearly impossible to find in their native habitats. Ask yourself the following questions before gathering:

◆ Is this plant endangered? If so, it may be illegal to gather it.

◆ Should this herb be taken from the wild for personal use, or can it be purchased or cultivated?

◆ What part of the plant do I need? In the US and Europe, the ginkgo's leaves are considered the medicinal portion of the ginkgo tree. Leaves are best gathered in late summer when their active compounds are at their most concentrated.

◆ What will I be using this herb for and exactly how much of it do I need?

◆ Is the ground wet where the tree is growing? If so, find trees growing in a dry spot or return when the ground is dry. Walking on wet soil compresses the dirt, making it difficult for future growth.

◆ Can I leave behind enough healthy leaves for the local animal population?

DO-IT-YOURSELF
REMEDIES

CAPSULE You can make your own herbal supplements by purchasing animal or vegetable gelatin capsules at your local health food store and packing each capsule with 40mg dried, powdered ginkgo leaves. Standard dosage: 40mg ginkgo extract three times daily.

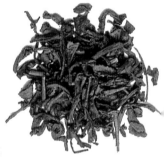

DRYING Wash, thoroughly dry, and chop fresh ginkgo leaves into small pieces. Lay the chopped herb on trays in a dry, well-ventilated, shaded area of your home, or place in an oven on a very low temperature, making sure air is continually circulating around the herbs, or use a dehydrator. Drying will take between seven and 14 days. When drying herbs either in a warm room or in an oven, the temperature should be kept between 20°–30°C (70°–90°F). Store the dried root in a dark, airtight, nonporous container.

FOMENTATION Fomentations are essentially gauze or surgical bandages soaked in freshly made herbal tea. The hot cloth is then laid directly on a bite, rash, or wound.

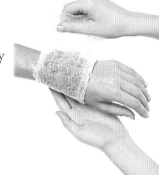

INFUSED OIL MADE WITH FRESH LEAVES

Infused oils boast the fat-soluble active principles of whatever medicinal plant or herb has been used to make them. One way to create ginkgo oil is to tightly pack a clean jar to its top with fresh ginkgo leaves. Pour almond or olive oil into the jar to cover the herb. Seal the jar tightly and leave in a warm place for six to seven weeks. Shake it daily. When ready to use, strain the oil and store in a dark, airtight container for up to two years. Infused oil can be ingested or used externally.

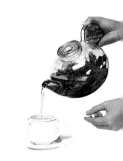

LIQUID EXTRACT Also known as extract. To make ginkgo extract, macerate 100-200g of dried ginkgo leaves, or 300-500g of fresh leaves. Place the herb in a jar and pour in 335ml vodka (40% alcohol by volume) and 165ml water. Screw the lid on the jar and store in a dark area for four to eight weeks. Shake the mixture daily. When ready, strain the mixture, pressing all remaining liquid from the ginkgo leaves. Place liquid in a nonreactive saucepan and simmer over medium heat for 20-40 minutes until the liquid has been reduced by a third. This process burns off the alcohol, leaving the medicinal liquid behind. Allow the liquid to cool and decant into several dropper bottles or a clean glass bottle. Will keep up to two years. Shake before using. Standard dosage: 5ml three times a day.

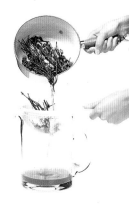

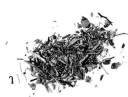

OINTMENT Also called a salve, herbal ointment is easy to make at home. To create your own ginkgo ointment, mix 1 to 2 parts beeswax or soft paraffin wax, 7 parts cocoa butter, and 3 parts dried, powdered ginkgo leaves in a nonreactive saucepan. Cook the mixture for one to two hours on a low setting. Leave to cool, package in an airtight container, and apply up to three times a day when required.

POULTICE Fresh herbs can be applied directly to the skin when fashioned into a poultice. To make a ginkgo poultice, chop the fresh or dried flowers and/or leaves. Boil in a small amount of water for five minutes (or use a microwave). Squeeze out any excess liquid from the boiled herb (reserve liquid). Lay the ginkgo leaves directly on to the skin and cover with a warm, moist towel. Leave in place for up to 30 minutes. The reserved liquid can be rewarmed.

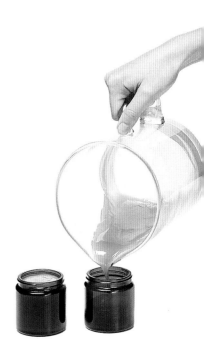

TEA Also known as an infusion, tea is an easy and common way to ingest an herb. To make ginkgo tea, steep 1 teaspoon of dried ginkgo leaves or 1 tablespoon fresh leaves for five minutes in a cup of boiling water. You may add fructose, sugar, or honey to sweeten. Standard dosage: 1 cup of tea three times daily.

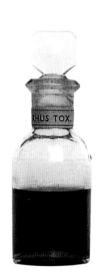

TINCTURES Though they are not as potent as liquid extracts, tinctures are minimally processed, making them a favourite remedy among herbalists. To make your own ginkgo tincture, place 100–200g of dried ginkgo leaves or 300–500g of fresh ginkgo leaves in a large jar and cover with 500ml vodka (40% alcohol by volume). Place the lid on the jar and store in a dark area for four to six weeks. Shake the bottle daily. When ready to use strain the mixture, pressing all remaining liquid from the leaves. Decant into several dropper bottles or a clean glass bottle. Will keep for up to a year.

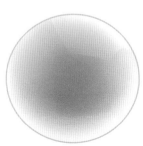

ALTERNATIVE HEALTH STRATEGIES

Herbs, vitamins, and minerals all contribute to good health. However, creating a sense of general well–being involves more than simply taking supplements. Health has to do with a quality of life that can often be aggravated by causes of harmful stress. Listed below are some additional ways to help keep yourself well.

IMPROVE YOUR EATING HABITS

Listed below are the five main eating strategies people follow; consider finding the healthiest one that suits your lifestyle.

- ◆ Omnivore
- ◆ Semi-vegetarian
- ◆ Macrobiotic
- ◆ Vegan
- ◆ Vegetarian

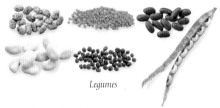

Legumes

GET MORE EXERCISE

Whether it's walking or weightlifting, any type of exercise can help you feel better. Try any of these types:

- ◆ Stretching
- ◆ Aerobics
- ◆ Resistance training

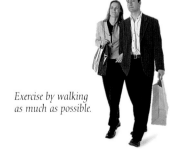

Exercise by walking as much as possible.

SIMPLE WAYS TO EASE STRESS

In addition to exercise and healthy eating, here are some more techniques – old and new – for easing stress and increasing relaxation.

◆ Get enough sleep
◆ Take time to relax
◆ Give up junk food
◆ Adopt a pet
◆ Surround yourself with supportive people
◆ Limit your exposure to chemicals
◆ Enjoy yourself

ᐧ ONE-MINUTE STRESS REDUCER ᐧ

Deep breathing can be done anywhere and anytime you need to calm and centre yourself:

1 Inhale deeply through your nose.
2 Hold your breath for up to three seconds, then exhale your breath through your mouth.
3 Continue as needed.

Deep breathing draws a person's attention away from a given stress and refocuses it on his or her breathing. This type of breathing is not only comforting (thanks to its rhythmic quality), but also has been shown to lower rapid pulse and shallow respiration – two temporary symptoms of stress.

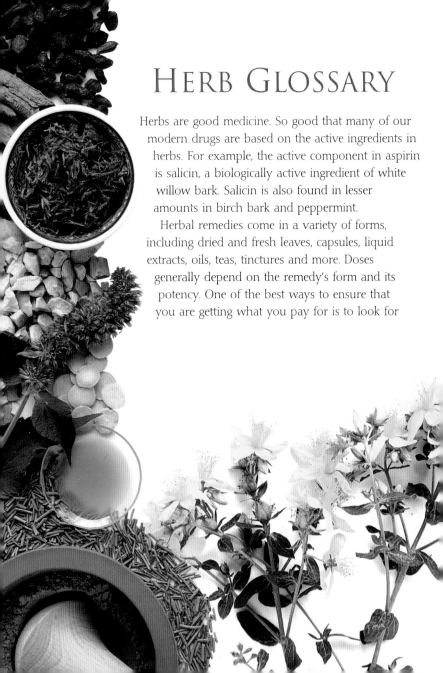

HERB GLOSSARY

Herbs are good medicine. So good that many of our modern drugs are based on the active ingredients in herbs. For example, the active component in aspirin is salicin, a biologically active ingredient of white willow bark. Salicin is also found in lesser amounts in birch bark and peppermint.

Herbal remedies come in a variety of forms, including dried and fresh leaves, capsules, liquid extracts, oils, teas, tinctures and more. Doses generally depend on the remedy's form and its potency. One of the best ways to ensure that you are getting what you pay for is to look for

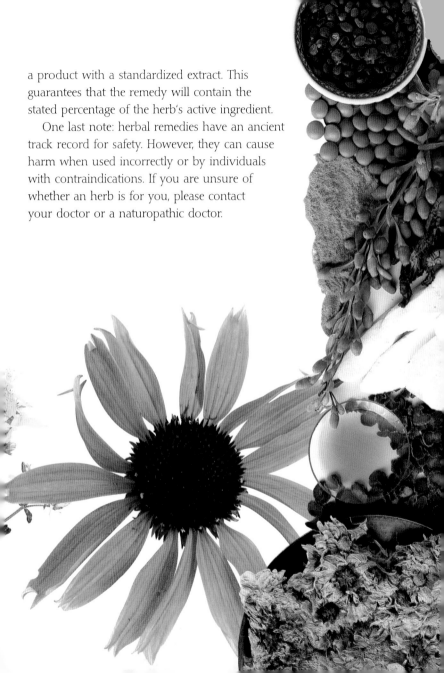

a product with a standardized extract. This guarantees that the remedy will contain the stated percentage of the herb's active ingredient.

One last note: herbal remedies have an ancient track record for safety. However, they can cause harm when used incorrectly or by individuals with contraindications. If you are unsure of whether an herb is for you, please contact your doctor or a naturopathic doctor.

ACHILLEA MILLEFOLIUM
Yarrow

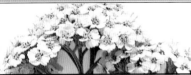

Properties Antibacterial, anti-inflammatory, antispasmodic, blood coagulator, bile stimulating, immune-system stimulant, promotes sweating, sedative.

Target Ailments Anxiety, colds and flu, cystitis, digestive disorders, menstrual cramps, minor wounds, nosebleeds, poor circulation, skin rashes.

Available Forms Dried herb, capsule, liquid extract, oil, tea, tincture.

Possible Side Effects Diarrhoea, skin rash.

Precautions Yarrow is related to ragweed and can cause an allergic reaction in individuals with ragweed allergies. Do not take if pregnant; it can induce miscarriage.

ALLIUM SATIVUM
Garlic

Properties Antibacterial, anticoagulant, antifungal, anti-inflammatory, antiviral, cholesterol reducer, digestive aid, immune-system stimulant, worm-fighting.

Target Ailments Arteriosclerosis, arthritis, bladder infections, colds, digestive upset, flu, heart conditions, high blood pressure, high blood cholesterol, viral infections.

Available Forms Capsule, fresh cloves, liquid extract, oil, tincture.

Possible Side Effects Can cause upset stomach.

Precautions While garlic is safe taken in culinary doses, individuals on anticoagulant medications should consult their doctor before supplementing their diet with garlic.

ASTRAGALUS SPP.
Astragalus

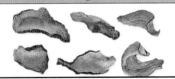

Properties Antibacterial, anti-inflammatory, antioxidant, antiviral, diuretic, immune-system stimulant.

Target Ailments Cancer, colds, appetite loss, diarrhoea, fatigue, flu, heart conditions, HIV, viral infections.

Available Forms Capsule, dried herb, fresh herb, liquid extract, tea, tincture.

Possible Side Effects None expected.

Precautions Astragalus should be used as a companion therapy to – not a replacement for – traditional cancer and HIV therapies.

CALENDULA OFFICINALIS
Calendula

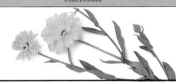

Properties Antibacterial, anti-inflammatory, antiseptic, antispasmodic, promotes sweating, sedative.

Target Ailments Burns, cuts, fungal infections, gallbladder conditions, hepatitis, indigestion, irregular menstruation, insect bites, menstrual cramps, mouth sores, skin rashes, ulcers, wounds.

Available Forms Capsule, dried herb, fresh herb, liquid extract, lotion, oil, ointment, tincture.

Possible Side Effects None expected.

Precautions Calendula is related to ragweed. Individuals allergic to ragweed should consult a doctor before using calendula.

ALOE VERA
Aloe

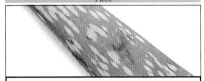

Properties Analgesic, antibacterial, antifungal, anti-inflammatory, anti-itch, antiseptic, circulatory stimulant, digestive aid, immune-system stimulant, laxative.

Target Ailments Acne, bruises, burns, constipation, cuts, insect bites, digestive disorders, rashes, ulcers, wounds.

Available Forms Capsule, fresh leaves, gel, juice, liquid extract.

Possible Side Effects When taken internally, aloe can cause severe cramping in some individuals.

Precautions Pregnant women should not ingest aloe; It can stimulate uterine contractions.

ANGELICA POLYMORPHA
Dong Quai

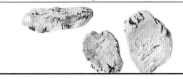

Properties Antiallergenic, antispasmodic, diuretic, mild laxative, muscle relaxant, vasodilator.

Target Ailments Abscesses, blurred vision, heart palpitations, irregular menstruation, light-headedness, menstrual pain, pallor, poor circulation.

Available Forms Capsule, dried herb, liquid extract, tincture.

Possible Side Effects Can cause photosensitivity in some individuals.

Precautions Dong quai has abortive abilities; Do not take while pregnant.

CHAMAEMELUM NOBILE
Chamomile

Properties Antibacterial, anti-inflammatory, antiseptic, antispasmodic, carminative, digestive aid, fever reducer, sedative.

Target Ailments Gingivitis, haemorrhoids, insomnia, indigestion, intestinal gas, menstrual cramps, nausea, nervousness, stomachaches, sunburns, tension, ulcers, varicose veins.

Available Forms Capsule, dried herb, fresh herb, liquid extract, lotion, oil, tea, tincture.

Possible Side Effects None expected.

Precautions Because chamomile is related to ragweed, individuals with ragweed allergies should consult a doctor before using chamomile.

DIOSCOREA VILLOSA
Wild Yam

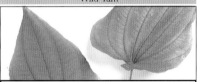

Properties Analgesic, anti-inflammatory, antispasmodic, expectorant, muscle relaxant, promotes sweating.

Target Ailments Menopause, menstrual cramps, morning sickness, nausea, rheumatoid arthritis, urinary tract infections.

Available Forms Capsule, cream, dried root, liquid extract, oil, powder, tincture.

Possible Side Effects Can cause vomiting in large doses.

Precautions Individuals who are suffering from a hormone-sensitive cancer, such as breast or uterine cancer, should avoid wild yam. Some experts believe that the herb can encourage the growth of cancer cells.

ECHINACEA PURPUREA
Echinacea

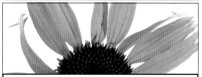

Properties Antiallergenic, antibacterial, antiseptic, antimicrobial, antiviral, carminative, lymphatic tonic.

Target Ailments Abscesses, acne, bladder infections, blood poisoning, burns, colds, eczema, food poisoning, flu, insect bites, kidney infections, mononucleosis, respiratory infections, sore throats.

Available Forms Capsule, dried herb, liquid extract, tea, tincture.

Possible Side Effects High doses can cause dizziness and nausea.

Precautions Do not take echinacea for more than four weeks in a row.

GINKGO BILOBA
Ginkgo

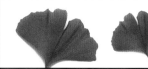

Properties Antibacterial, anti-inflammatory, antioxidant, circulatory stimulant, vasodilator.

Target Ailments Clotting disorders, dementia, depression, headaches, hearing loss, Raynaud's syndrome, tinnitus, vascular diseases, vertigo.

Available Forms Capsule, dry herb, liquid extract, tincture, tea.

Possible Side Effects Diarrhoea, irritability, nausea, restlessness.

Precautions Do not use ginkgo biloba if you have a blood-clotting disorder like haemophilia or are taking anticoagulant medications.

LAVANDULA SPP.
Lavender

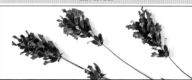

Properties Antibacterial, antidepressant, antiseptic, antispasmodic, carminative, circulatory stimulant, digestive aid, diuretic, sedative.

Target Ailments Anxiety, depression, headache, insomnia, intestinal gas, nausea, tension.

Available Forms Capsule, dried herb, fresh herb, oil, tincture.

Possible Side Effects Lavender products can cause skin irritation in sensitive individuals.

Precautions Lavender oil is poisonous when ingested internally.

MENTHA PIPERITA
Peppermint

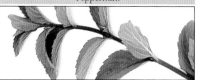

Properties Antacid, antibacterial, antidepressant, antispasmodic, carminatve, expectorant, muscle relaxant, promotes sweating.

Target Ailments Anxiety, colds, fever, flu, insomnia, intestinal gas, itching, migraines, morning sickness, motion sickness, nausea.

Available Forms Capsule, dried herb, fresh herb, lozenge, oil, ointment, tea, tincture.

Possible Side Effects When applied externally, peppermint products can cause skin reactions in sensitive individuals.

Precautions If you have a hiatal hernia, talk to your doctor before using peppermint products externally or internally; the oil in the plant can exacerbate symptoms.

HYDRASTIS CANADENSIS
Goldenseal

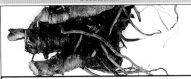

Properties Antacid, antibacterial, antifungal, anti-inflammatory, antiseptic, astringent, digestive aid, stimulant.

Target Ailments Canker sores, contact dermatitis, diarrhoea, eczema, food poisoning. **Available Forms** Capsule, dry herb, liquid extract, tea, tincture.

Possible Side Effects In high doses, goldenseal can cause diarrhoea and nausea and can irritate the skin, mouth and throat.

Precautions Because of its high cost, many manufacturers adulterate preparations with less costly herbs, such as barberry, yellow dock or bloodroot, some of which can cause unwanted reactions when taken in high doses.

HYPERICUM PERFORATUM
St John's wort

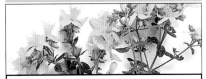

Properties Analgesic, antibacterial, anti-depressant, anti-inflammatory, antiviral, astringent.

Target Ailments Attention deficit disorder, anxiety, bacterial infections, burns, carpal tunnel syndrome, depression. menopause.

Available Forms Capsule, dried herb, liquid extract, oil, ointment, tea, tincture.

Possible Side Effects Gastrointestinal upset, headaches, photosensitivity, stiff neck.

Precautions Avoid foods containing the amino acid tyramine when taking St John's wort; the interaction of the two can cause an increase in blood pressure. Foods with tyramine include beer, coffee, wine, chocolate and fava beans.

PENAX SPP.
Ginseng

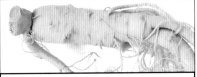

Properties Antibacterial, antidepressant, immune-system stimulant, stimulant.

Target Ailments Colds, depression, fatigue, flu, impaired immune system, respiratory conditions, stress.

Available Forms Capsule, dried root, fresh root, liquid extract, tincture, tea.

Possible Side Effects Large doses of ginseng can cause breast soreness, headaches or skin rashes in some individuals.

Precautions Ginseng can aggravate existing heart palpitations or high blood pressure.

PETROSELINUM CRISPUM
Parsley

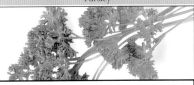

Properties Antiseptic, antispasmodic, digestive aid, diuretic, laxative, muscle relaxant.

Target Ailments Colds, congestion, fever, flu, indigestion, irregular menstruation, premenstrual syndrome, stimulating the production of breast milk, stomachaches.

Available Forms Capsule, dried herb, fresh herb, liquid extract, oil, tea, tincture.

Possible Side Effects Can cause photosensitivity in some individuals.

Precautions Parsley should not be ingested in large amounts or used externally during pregnancy; it contains compounds that may stimulate uterine muscles and possibly cause miscarriage.

PIPER METHYSTICUM
Kava

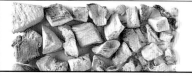

Properties Antidepressant, antispasmodic, aphrodisiac, diuretic, muscle relaxant, sedative.

Target Ailments Anxiety, colds, depression, menstrual conditions, muscle cramps, respiratory tract conditions, stress.

Available Forms Capsule, dried herb, liquid extract, tea, tincture.

Possible Side Effects Allergic skin reactions, muscle weakness, red eyes, sleepiness.

Precautions In high doses, kava can impair motor reflexes and cause breathing problems.

ROSMARINUS OFFICINALIS
Rosemary

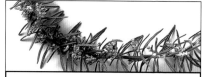

Properties Antibacterial, antidepressant, anti-inflammatory, antiseptic, carminative, circulatory stimulant.

Target Ailments Bad breath, dandruff, depression, eczema, headaches, indigestion, joint inflammation, mouth and throat infections, muscle pain, psoriasis, rheumatoid arthritis.

Available Forms Dried herb, fresh herb, ingestible rosemary-flavoured oil, oil, ointment, tea, tincture.

Possible Side Effects Rosemary oil can cause skin inflammation and/or dermatitis.

Precautions Do not mistake regular rosemary oil for ingestible rosemary-flavoured oil.

SILYBUM
Milk Thistle

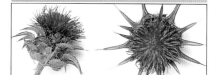

Properties Anti-inflammatory, antioxidant, digestive aid, immune-system stimulant.

Target Ailments Inflammation of the gall-bladder duct, hepatitis, liver conditions, poisoning from ingestion of the death cup mushroom, psoriasis.

Available Forms Capsule, dried herb, fresh herb, powder, tea, tincture.

Possible Side Effects Milk thistle can cause mild diarrhoea when taken in large doses.

Precautions If you think you have a liver disorder, seek medical advice before taking this herb.

TANACETUM PARTHENIUM
Feverfew

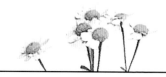

Properties Anti-inflammatory, fever reducer.

Target Ailments Arthritis, asthma, dermatitis, menstrual pain, migraines.

Available Forms Capsule, dried herb, fresh herb, liquid extract, tincture.

Possible Side Effects Some individuals experience "withdrawal" symptoms after taking feverfew, including fatigue and nervousness.

Precautions Because it is related to ragweed, individuals with ragweed allergies should consult a doctor before using feverfew.

SALVIA SPP
Sage

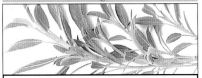

Properties Antiseptic, anti-inflammatory, antioxidant, antispasmodic, astringent, bile stimulant, carminative, reduces perspiration.

Target Ailments Excess intestinal gas, insect bites, menopausal night sweats, poor circulation, reduces milk flow at weaning, sore throat, stomachaches, mouth ulcers.

Available Forms Capsule, dried herb, fresh herb, liquid extract, oil, tincture.

Possible Side Effects Sage tea may cause inflammation of the lips and/or tongue in some individuals.

Precautions Do not ingest pure sage oil; it is toxic when taken internally.

SERENOA REPENS
Saw Palmetto

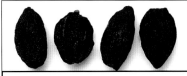

Properties Antiallergenic, anti-inflammatory, diuretic, immune-boosting.

Target Ailments Asthma, benign prostatic hyperplasia, bronchitis, colds, cystitis, impotence, male infertility, nasal congestion, sinus conditions, sore throats.

Available Forms Capsule, dried herb, fresh herb, liquid extract, oil, tea, tincture.

Possible Side Effects Can cause diarrhoea if taken in large doses.

Precautions Due to its hormonal actions, saw palmetto may interact negatively with prostate medicines or hormonal treatments such as oestrogen replacement therapy, possibly cancelling out their effectiveness.

VALERIANA OFFICINALIS
Valerian

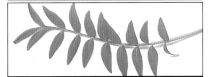

Properties Analgesic, antibacterial, antispasmodic, carminative, reduces blood pressure, sedative, tranquilizer.

Target Ailments Brachial spasm, high blood pressure, insomnia, palpitations, menstrual pain, migraines, muscle cramps, nervousness, tension headaches, wounds.

Available Forms Capsules, dried herb, liquid extract, oil, teas, tincture.

Possible Side Effects Headaches with prolonged use.

Precautions Do not take with other sedatives, including alcohol. Do not drive or operate machinery after taking valerian.

ZINGIBER OFFICINALE
Ginger

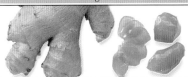

Properties Antibacterial, anticoagulant, antinausea, antispasmodic, antiviral, carminative, digestive aid, expectorant, immune-system stimulant, muscle relaxant.

Target Ailments Burns, colds, flu, high blood pressure, high cholesterol, liver conditions, intestinal gas, menstrual cramps, motion sickness, nausea, stomachaches.

Available Forms Capsule, dried root, tea.

Possible Side Effects Heartburn.

Precautions While ginger is safe in culinary doses, individuals who suffer from a blood-clotting disorder or are on anticoagulant medication should consult a physician before supplementing their diet with the herb.

HERBAL TERMS

ADAPTOGENIC Increases resistance and resilience to stress. Supports adrenal gland functioning.

ALTERATIVE Blood purifier that improves the condition of the blood, improves digestion, and increases the appetite. Used to treat conditions arising from or causing toxicity.

ANALGESIC HERB that relieves pain either by relaxing muscles or reducing pain signals to the brain.

ANTHELMINTIC Destroys or expels intestinal worms.

ANTACID Neutralizes excess stomach and intestinal acids.

ANTIALLERGENIC Inactivates allergenic substances in the body.

ANTIBACTERIAL/ANTIBIOTIC Helps the body fight off harmful bacteria.

ANTIDEPRESSANT Helps maintain emotional stability.

ANTICATARRHAL Eliminates or counteracts the formation of mucus.

ANTICOAGULANT Thins blood and helps prevent blood clots.

ANTIFUNGAL Kills infection-causing fungi.

ANTI-INFLAMMATORY Reduces swelling of the tissues.

ANTI-ITCH Deadens itching sensations.

ANTIMICROBIAL Kills a wide range of harmful bacteria, fungi, and viruses.

ANTIOXIDANT Fights harmful oxidation.

ANTIPYRETIC/FEVER REDUCER Reduces or prevents fever.

ANTISEPTIC External application prevents bacterial growth on skin.

ANTISPASMODIC Prevents or relaxes muscle tension.

ANTIVIRAL Helps the body fight invading viruses.

ASTRINGENT Has a constricting or binding effect. Commonly used to treat haemorrhages, secretions and diarrhoea.

BLOOD COAGULANT Thickens blood and aids in clotting.

CARMINATIVE Relieves gas.

CHOLAGOGUE Encourages the flow of bile into the small intestine.

CIRCULATORY STIMULANT Promotes even and efficient blood circulation.

DEMULCENT Soothing substance, usually mucilage, taken internally to protect injured or inflamed tissues.

DIAPHORETIC Induces sweating.

DIURETIC Increases urine flow.

EMETIC Induces vomiting.

EMMENAGOGUE Promotes menstruation.

EMOLLIE Softens, soothes and protects skin.

EXPECTORANT Assists in expelling mucus from the lungs and throat.

GALACTOGOGUE Increases the secretion of breast milk.

HEMOSTATIC Stops haemorrhaging and encourages blood coagulation.

HEPATIC Tones and strengthens the liver.

HYPOTENSIVE Lowers abnormally elevated blood pressure.

IMMUNE-SYSTEM STIMULANT Strengthens immune system so the body can fight off invading organisms.

LAXATIVE Promotes bowel movements.

LITHOTRIPTIC Helps dissolve urinary and biliary stones.

MUSCLE RELAXANT Loosens tight muscles and reduces muscle cramping.

NERVINE Calms tension.

OXYTOCIC Stimulates uterine contractions.

RUBEFACIENT Increases blood flow at the surface of the skin.

SEDATIVE Quiets the nervous system.

SIALAGOGUE/DIGESTIVE AID Promotes the flow of saliva.

STIMULANT Increases the body's energy.

TONIC Promotes the functions of body systems.

VASOCONSTRICTOR Constricts blood vessels, limiting the amount of blood flowing to a particular area.

VASODILATOR Dilates blood vessels, helping to promote blood flow.

VULNERARY Encourages wound healing by promoting cell growth and repair.

USEFUL ADDRESSES

PROFESSIONAL ASSOCIATIONS

Ayurvedic Living
PO Box 188,
Exeter,
Devon EX4 5AB

British Herbal Medicine Association
Sun House,
Church St,
Stroud GL5 1JL

European Herbal Practitioners Association
Midsummer Cottage,
Nether, Westcote,
Kingham, Oxon OX7 6SD

European Scientific Cooperative for Phytotherapy
Argyll House, Gandy St,
Exeter EX4 3LS

National Institute of Medical Herbalists
56 Longbrook Street,
Exeter EX4 6AH

Register of Chinese Herbal Medicine
PO Box 400
Wembley HA9 9NZ

TRAINING COURSES

Middlesex University
Queensway, Enfield,
Middlesex EN3 4SF

School of Phytotherapy
Bucksteep Manor,
Bodle Street Green,
Nr Hailsham,
East Sussex BN27 4RH

University of Central Lancashire
Preston PR1 2HE

University of Westminster
309 Regent St,
London W1

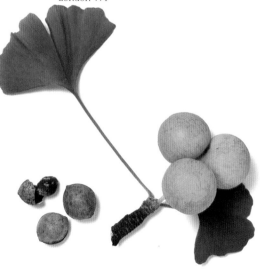

Herbal Suppliers

Western Herbs

Baldwin, G. & Co.
171–173 Walworth Road,
London SE17 1RW

Bio-Health Ltd (herbal capsules)
Culpeper Close,
Medway City Industrial Estate
Rochester ME2 4HU

Brome & Schimmer Ltd
Unit 42, Romsey Industrial Estate, Romsey,
Hants SO51 OHR

Culpeper Ltd (Head Office)
Hadstock Road, Linton,
Cambridge CB1 6NJ

East–West Herbs Ltd
Langston Priory Mews,
Kingham, Oxon OX7 6HP

East West Herb Shop
3 Neal's Yard,
London WC2H 9DP

Granary Herbs
The Granary, Bearsted,
Kent ME14 4NN

Hambledon Herbs
Court Farm, Milverton,
Somerset TA4 1NF

The Herbal Apothecary
103 High Street,
Syston, Leics LE7 1GQ

Napier & Sons
148 Dunbarton Road,
Edinburgh EH1 1EZ, and
1 Byres Road,
Glasgow GL11 6XE

Neal's Yard Remedies
15 Neal's Yard, Covent Garden,
London WC2H 9DP, and
Chelsea Farmers Market,
Sydney Street,
London SW3 6NR

Phytoproducts
Parkworks, Park Road, Mansfield
Woodhouse, Notts NG19 8EF

Potters Herbal Supplies
Leyland Mill Lane,
Wigan, Lancs WN1 2SB

Eastern Herbs

AcuMedic Centre
101–103 Camden High Street,
London NW1 7JN

East–West Herbs Ltd
East West Herb Shop
(see Western Herbs)

Mayway Herbal Emporium
43 Waterside Trading Centre,
Trumper's Way,
Hanwell W7 2Q

INDEX

ACKNOWLEDGEMENTS

DORLING 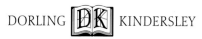 KINDERSLEY

LONDON, NEW YORK, SYDNEY, DEHLI, PARIS,
MUNICH, and JOHANNESBURG

Stephanie Pedersen is an American writer and editor who specializes in the
area of health. Her articles have appeared in numerous publications and she
has also co-written several books published by St. Martin's Press.

The publisher would like to thank Norma McGough BSc Hons FRD for
acting as UK consultant on the series.

....

Editorial Director: LaVonne Carlson
Editors: Nancy Burke, Barbara Minton, Connie Robinson
Designer: Carol Wells
Cover Designer: Gus Yoo

Picture Credits: Steve Gorton, David Murray, Dave King, Martin Norris,
Philip Gatward, Andy Crawford, Philip Dowell, Clive Streeter, Peter Chadwick,
Tim Ridley, Andrew Whittack, Martin Cameron

Copyright © 2001 Dorling Kindersley Limited

First published in Great Britain in 2001 by
Dorling Kindersley Limited
9 Henrietta Street, London, WC2E 8PS

2 4 6 8 10 9 7 5 3

A CIP catalogue record for this book is available from the British Library

ISBN 0 7513 31619

Reproduction by Dai Nippon Printing Co., (HK Ltd.)
Printed and bound in China by L.Rex Printing Co., Ltd.

see our complete catalogue at
www.dk.com